ADEENA WEISS

The Can't Sleep Solution Guide

30 Practical Tips to Help You Sleep to Improve your Physical and Mental Health

This book was professionally typeset on Reedsy.
Find out more at reedsy.com

Contents

Introduction

Getting the proper amount of high quality sleep is probably one of the most important health habits out there to maintain one's physical, emotional and mental health. Despite this, 1 in 5 people move through their day in a sleep-deprived state on a regular basis, and it is estimated that 1 in 10 people will develop chronic insomnia. This guide will briefly explain why sleep is so important, and then provide a whole bunch of practical tips which you can use to help you fall asleep and stay asleep, hopefully having you wake up refreshed, relaxed and energized!

My name is Adeena Weiss and I am a Physical Therapist, an ICF Certified Life Coach, and a COPE (Center for Obesity Prevention and Education) Certified Health and Wellness Coach. I wrote this book because good sleep habits were always something that eluded me. Despite knowing all the information, and helping my clients develop their healthy habits (of which sleep was quite up there in terms of importance), it was the one thing that I pretty much ignored for myself. I loved staying up late and working or reading or just fooling around on my phone well into the night. I rationalized that that quiet time of day (night!) was my "me time", and that since I was able to wake up on time, and go about my day energetic and in a good mood, I obviously don't need as much sleep as others and my crazy schedule works for me. And it did work.......until it didn't! A few years ago, something triggered a rare autoimmune disorder in my body, and in an effort to do all the things to decrease inflammation, I realized it was time to improve my sleep habits. In studying the best ways to help a person who doesn't/can't sleep learn to fall asleep and stay asleep, I've compiled a list of 30+ tips and strategies that research has shown to be helpful and effective.

Don't try to implement all 30+ at once! I always teach my clients that if you try to take on too much at once it can become overwhelming and unsustainable. My recommendation is to start off with one or two of the recommendations for a few nights. See how you feel. Do you notice improvement? Add on another one or two, and slowly build a healthy sleep routine! Everyone's body is different and what does the trick for one person might not be effective enough for another, so keep at it until you find what works for you. Make sure to give things a few nights for your body to adjust to the new routine, and for your habitual sleep cycle to adjust.

So now let's help you fall asleep easily and stay asleep for the amount of time your body needs to be its best!

1

Am I Sleeping Enough?

How do I know if I'm getting enough sleep?

The American Academy of Sleep Medicine and the Sleep Research Society recommend adults sleep at least 7-8 hours a night. However, everyone's body is different and some people require more than that to feel energized and thriving, while others seem to do very well with less. Here are some questions you can ask yourself to know if you are getting enough sleep, and/ or if the sleep you are getting is of poor quality. You can check off any and all that apply to you.

- Do you wake up feeling tired and lacking energy?
- Do you hit the snooze button numerous times before you can get out of bed?
- Do you have a tendency to oversleep?
- Do you fall asleep with the TV on or while reading?
- Are you unable to function without a coffee in the morning?

- Do you need a coffee, cola, or energy drinks during the day to keep you going?
- Do you need a nap in the middle of the day in order to make it through the day?
- Do you have trouble focusing throughout the day? How's your memory? Your attention?
- Do you find yourself craving carbs and use the carbs to have sufficient energy to get through the day?
- Are you irritable and grumpy? Moody? Unmotivated?
- Are you feeling draggy or unproductive?
- Do you need to drink alcohol to get to sleep?
- Do you need to take sleeping pills to get to sleep?
- Do you eat large and carbohydrate filled meals in the evening?
- Does it take you a long time to fall asleep?
- Do you wake frequently in the night? Do you have a hard time getting back to sleep?
- Do you wake up too early and can't get back to sleep?

If you have a number of these checked off, it's likely that you are either not sleeping enough for your body's needs, or the sleep you are getting is of poor quality. Please note that for some of these questions there can be other causes of these symptoms (things such as sleep apnea, hypothyroidism,hormonal imbalance, depression, anxiety disorder) so if you suspect something else is going on in your body in addition to the sleep deprivation, or if you are consistently utilizing good sleep habits and following the tips but are not seeing improvement, please consult with your doctor to rule out any physical or mental health causes.

2

What Triggers Insomnia?

Why can't I sleep?

There are two types of insomnia- which is difficulty with either falling asleep at night, or difficulty staying asleep. The first type is a short term or Acute Insomnia which can last for a few days or even up to a number of weeks and in some cases, a few months. Up to 50% of adults will experience this at some point in their lives, and it is often due to situational stress or a stressful incident. It can also be set off by changes in your schedule, major life events or transitions, time zone changes or jet lag. Pain, such as from an injury or surgery, or discomfort from a short term illness might be another cause of short term insomnia. Changes in, or side effects of medications can also contribute. And at times, the trigger behind the insomnia is unknown. Acute Insomnia is often self limiting, but in a percentage of people it may become a chronic condition.

The second type of insomnia is a long term or Chronic Insomnia, which is difficulty sleeping at least 3 times a week for over 3 months. This type of insomnia can even last years, and can have many adverse ramifications on a person's health and well-being. It's estimated that up to 10% of the population struggles with Chronic Insomnia! That's crazy! We are definitely a sleep deprived society.

It is important to note that although insomnia can be a primary problem, it can also be secondary to, or a symptom of, other medical or psychological conditions, so any new pattern of insomnia in which no cause can be pinpointed should be brought up to a medical professional in order to rule out a medical cause that would require intervention (examples might be things like Sleep Apnea or Clinical Depression).

Here are some things which can be causing your chronic sleeplessness-

- Stress, like with Acute Insomnia, is probably the most frequent reason people struggle with Chronic Insomnia. Worry and anxiety about life events such as difficulties with one's children, death or illness of a loved one, troublesome world events, divorce, worries about one's health, finances or job are all stressors that could set off a pattern of sleeplessness that can become chronic. Mental health disorders such as Depression, Post-Traumatic Stress Disorder or Chronic Anxiety also can often disrupt sleep patterns.

- Poor sleep habits can also be a cause of chronic difficulty in sleeping. Trying to sleep in an uncomfortable physical environment, going to sleep and waking at irregular times or sleeping too much during the day, or utilizing caffeine and other stimulants are all things which can make it difficult to fall asleep. Utilizing alcohol to sleep might initially help you fall asleep, but it stops you from getting into the deeper stages of sleep which you need for mental and physical health, and is likely to make you wake up in the middle of the night.

- As mentioned before, medical conditions can often cause sleeplessness either due to pain, due to side effects of the condition, or even due to side effects from medications given to treat the condition. Examples are GERD (reflux/heartburn), heart conditions, hormonal conditions, diabetes, respiratory conditions like asthma, cancer, and degenerative brain diseases such as Alzheimers or Parkinsons. Other conditions affecting sleep are Restless Leg Syndrome, muscle spasms, and sleep apnea-in which a person has brief episodes of stopping breathing while they are sleeping. Mental health disorders such as Depression, Post-Traumatic Stress Disorder or Chronic Anxiety also can often disrupt sleep patterns.

- Another factor might be one's evening eating habits. Dense or high fat meals during dinner, or eating right before going to sleep forces the body into working on digestion instead of winding down. Eating a lot before bedtime can make you uncomfortable lying down and can cause or exacerbate reflux or heartburn which can be painful and make it difficult to sleep.

- Changes to your work schedule or travel to different time zones can interfere with your sleep cycle and disrupt the circadian rhythm , which is your internal clock.

- Some medications such as blood pressure medications, asthma medication and some antidepressants have sleeplessness as a possible side effect. In addition, there are many over the counter medications and natural supplements that can contain stimulants such as caffeine that can also interfere with your ability to sleep. Examples may be weight loss supplements, cold/allergy medications, and pain medications.

- Many people develop sleep issues as they age due to changes in circadian rhythm (the internal clock moves forward causing one to get tired earlier, and wake up earlier), decreases in physical activity and/or social and mental stimulation causing increased napping during the day, pain due to physical conditions such as arthritis, increased use of prescription medications, and an increased need to urinate during the night due to bladder or prostate problems.

- Women are at increased risk of developing difficulty sleeping due to hormonal changes during the menstrual cycle and pregnancy, and during menopause due to hot flashes and night sweats.

3

Why is Sleep So Important?

What is the problem with sleep deprivation?

Sleep deprivation can have numerous adverse effects on both one's physical and mental health, ability to function at optimal levels, and on one's quality of life.

A major factor is the change in hormone levels that are disrupted by inadequate sleep which affects many functions of the body:

- Human Growth Hormone is only released during deep sleep and is in charge of cell growth and repair. Deficiency in this hormone affects our ability for protein production and synthesis, muscle development, metabolism, and natural immunity.

- Decreased sleep interrupts the levels of Leptin, Ghrelin, and Insulin, which are the hormones that regulate metabolism and are responsible for one's hunger signals, sense of fullness, blood sugar regulation and fat storage. Therefore, not getting enough sleep makes one hungrier, increases cravings and carbohydrate intake, and increases the chances of developing insulin resistance and diabetes! It is very difficult to lose weight if one is not sleeping properly.

- Poor sleep also affects the production of Melatonin which in turn affects the sleep cycle in the brain- therefore creating an increased vicious cycle of sleep disorder. In addition to Melatonin affecting your ability to sleep, lack of enough Melatonin also affects the working of hundreds of genes in the body.

- Poor sleep causes an increase in the stress hormone Cortisol in the body. Cortisol regulates other hormones in the body, and abnormal changes in cortisol levels affects the release of hormones such as Thyroid Hormone and Estrogen. In addition, increased Cortisol is one of the major causes of inflammation and inflammatory conditions in the body, and increased inflammation can cause or exacerbate autoimmune diseases, cancers, heart disease, high blood pressure, thyroid disease, and diabetes.

So you can see how severely a lack of sleep can affect our physical health, by causing spikes in appetite and weight gain, and increased inflammation and decreased immunity which leads to increased infections, illness and disease.

In addition to the numerous physical health ramifications, due to decreased time in the REM stage of sleep (Rapid-Eye-Movement phase of sleep, the deep phase of sleep when we dream), there are numerous effects on our mental and emotional health which can challenge our ability to function at optimal levels and show up in the way we want to show up.

- It can exacerbate mental health conditions such as depression and anxiety as well as addictions such as alcohol abuse.

- Sleeplessness will cause someone to feel a sense of tiredness, lack of energy, lack of motivation, and leave one with a general feeling of being unwell.

- It can cause increased grumpiness or moodiness which can have impact on one's interpersonal relationships

- It can cause an increase in behavioral issues such as aggressive behavior, lack of impulse control and hyperactivity.

- It can affect one's memory, ability to process information and learn new things, affecting one's performance in school or on the job.

- Not having sufficient sleep can cause a slowdown in one's thought process, increased clumsiness and decreased reaction times, which can cause an increase in car accidents.

As you can see, getting sufficient sleep on a regular basis can have numerous benefits: More energy, better mood, improved mental function, improved immunity, decreased inflammation, decreased risk of heart disease, balanced hormones, improved muscle recovery and cellular repair, decreased stress and decreased weight!

So I would venture to say that it's worthwhile to try to improve our sleep habits!

4

What Can I Do To Sleep Better??

30 + tips for for better sleep

It's all well and good to understand why we need more sleep, but how can we get that much needed 7–8 hours if our bodies and minds won't cooperate?

I've compiled a list of over 30 researched tips and tricks to help make it easier to fall asleep and stay asleep. Hopefully over time, you can incorporate as many of these as possible into your routine, and cause a big difference in your ability to sleep.

Tip #1

Have a Routine for sleep time and wake up time

Have your alarm go off at the same time every day in the morning, and go to sleep at the same time every day (early enough to be able to get at least 7 hours of uninterrupted sleep). And by every day, I do mean every single day, including weekends and vacations. According to the Mayo Clinic, changing your routine confuses your biological clock and stops it from getting and staying in a proper cycle.

When your alarm rings, get out of bed right away, don't press snooze. If you find yourself dependent on the snooze button, or if you find you can't get up on the weekends, it's an indication that you are not getting enough quality sleep. If you have difficulty getting up to an alarm, try using a dawn simulator, which is a light that you preset to gradually get brighter and brighter, like a sun rising. This causes the brain to start producing melatonin (which doesn't just put you to sleep- it regulates your sleep/ wake cycle), and it gets your body prepared to wake up more naturally.

Tip #2

Decrease the caffeine

I'm not saying not to have a morning coffee if you enjoy it, but make sure not to have any coffee by the time the afternoon rolls around, and make sure not to have any products at all that contain caffeine within 3 hours of going to bed, including green or black teas, sodas or chocolate. I know, we all love our chocolate, but if sleep is a problem, caffeine in the evening will exacerbate the issue. Caffeine is a strong (and addictive) stimulant, and its effects can last up to 8 hours, causing your body and mind to have difficulty settling down.

Tip #3

Watch what you are eating in the evening

Although the latest research seems to say that a light, nutrient rich snack is fine before bedtime, eating a large, heavy or fatty meal in the evening causes the body to have to work on digestion rather than other things it should be doing such as repair. It can also make it uncomfortable to lie down, and can cause reflux, heartburn, weight gain, and worse sleep. It is recommended that dinner be no closer than 2- 4 hours before bedtime to improve sleep. Keep in mind that a balanced diet throughout the day, incorporating whole grains, lean meats, fruits and vegetables has also shown evidence that it supports improved sleep.

Tip #4

Choose the right time to exercise

Exercise is fantastic for our bodies. 20 minutes of exercise in the morning can energize you, improve your mood and your focus for up to 12 hours. It can actually increase the chemicals in the body that can improve sleep, and is highly recommended. However, for most people, exercising right before bed is way too stimulating and can keep you awake. Avoid exercising for at least 4 hours before going to bed (aside for some calming yoga moves or tai chi to relax)

Tip #5

Use natural light to reset

30 minutes of natural light in the morning can reset your Circadian Rhythm and get you into a good cycle for better ability to fall asleep at night. Go outside in the morning or open the shades and let the light shine in. If you live in an area where there is not a lot of natural light, or it's often overcast, you can use a lightbox for some light therapy. Make sure that you get the box only from a reputable manufacturer, or from your dermatologist (they use it for skin conditions). It simulates natural light and can help adjust your cycle just as sunlight can.

Tip #6

Avoid alcohol

Alcohol suppresses the normal sleep pattern and should be avoided for at least 3 hours before bedtime. Although it can make you fall asleep faster, as it's being processed by the body it fragments your sleep by disrupting the ability to get into the deeper stages of the sleep cycle, and can cause you to wake up in the middle of the night, decreasing your body's ability to get quality sleep.

Tip #7

Avoid cigarettes and other stimulants

The nicotine in cigarettes is a stimulant, just like caffeine is. Smoking near bedtime will cause a release of hormones that increases a person's breathing rate, blood pressure, and heart rate. This will make it hard to fall asleep and can cause a person to wake up during the night, not allowing them to achieve a good quality and uninterrupted sleep.

Tip #8

Beware of the nap

Although there are mood and productivity benefits to power napping early in the afternoon, napping too late in the day will stop you from feeling tired at bedtime and make it hard to fall asleep. Make sure that naps take place at least 8 hours before you plan to go to sleep, and that they are for no longer than 20 minutes in duration.

Tip #9

Keep a sleep diary

Keeping daily track of your sleep times, nighttime wakefulness, and your habits surrounding your sleep will bring awareness of patterns that may be affecting your sleep. It is often recommended by doctors when someone comes to them complaining of an inability to sleep. A sleep diary or log will often include things like bedtimes, wake-up times, length of time it takes to fall asleep, how many sleep interruptions there were and how long they lasted, the number and duration of daytime naps, the perceived quality of sleep, how much alcohol, caffeine, or cigarettes was used during the day, the medications that were used, and what type and how much exercise was done. It can give a good overall picture of what's going on and help yourself or your doctor pinpoint things that may be affecting your sleep.

Tip #10

Destress near bedtime with calming activities

Clearing your mind of the day's anxieties can help you settle down both your body and your mind. Ideas to help destress include yoga, meditating, progressive relaxation, Tai Chi, journaling, deep breathing, reading (make sure to set a time limit!), or listening to calming ambient music.

Tip #11

Wind down the electronics

As it gets closer to bedtime, start winding down by dimming the lights, and at least an hour before bedtime shut the TV, laptop and phone. Stop emailing, and stop scrolling on the internet. Electronics emit "blue light" which messes with your circadian rhythm and sleep cycle by suppressing the body's production of Melatonin. In addition, the electronics are addictive, stimulating and distracting which tends to engage us for way longer than anticipated and can seriously cut into our sleep time.

Tip #12

Keep the cellphone out of the bedroom altogether

Aside from the blue light and the distraction factor, the texts and notifications can cause noise and vibration which can interrupt sleep. Even worse, cell phones also put out radiation which stimulates the brain. Research shows that people who use their phones at night get more headaches and have more difficulty falling asleep. If you do use your phone in the evening, shut it off at least 2 hours before bedtime, and preferably use headphones rather than holding it to your ear.

Tip #13

Lose the clutter

Sleeping in a clean, organized space will help you get a better quality sleep. Visual clutter can consciously or subconsciously cause a sense of stress or anxiety, which makes it psychologically harder to relax. Clearing it up also decreases visual distraction and decreasing our sensory input helps us fall asleep faster. In addition, a decluttered space is easier to keep clean and dust-free, which improves our air quality. This directly impacts our breathing, and therefore, our sleep. Try a 5 minute cleanup before beginning the nightly wind-down routine, to be ready to fully relax once you lay down.

Tip #14

Decrease liquid intake before bed

Many people wake up at night, sometimes numerous times, because of the need to go to the bathroom. If this is an issue for you, try stopping drinking anything within 2 hours of bedtime, and make sure to use the bathroom right before you go to bed.

Tip #15

Try meditation

Take a few minutes to focus on the present and bring your body into a calm, centered state. The meditation actually can lower your blood pressure and heart rate and slow down your breathing, which puts your body already into a sleeplike state. You can use audio guided meditations that can help calm your mind from constant intrusive thoughts and anxiety provoking thoughts from your busy day.

Tip #16

Focus on calm breathing

It's important to not only take 5 minutes to destress right before bed, but to take the time and notice stress building during the day, so you can utilize calming practices in the moment. That way stressful thoughts don't accumulate and haunt you at night. Focused and purposeful breathing is a great way to quickly bring your body into a calmer state. Here's one deep breathing practice that can be used to de-stress, both during the day during stressful moments, and at night to calm yourself down to sleep.

Take a deep centering breath. Then inhale for 6 seconds, hold it for 2 seconds, and exhale for 7 seconds. Do this a few times and you will feel the stress dissipate with each exhale.

Tip #17

Create a regular nighttime ritual

Take a few of the suggestions in this book, or anything else that suits you and your life, and create a regular nightly ritual that will signal your body that it is time to wind down. After a few nights of consistent ritual, your brain will automatically start associating sleep with the activities you are doing.

An example might be taking the dog for a short walk, dimming the lights and shutting electronics, spend 5 minutes tidying your sleep space/ preparing your room, get in cozy pajamas, use the bathroom, brush your teeth, get into bed, shut the light, do 5 minutes of meditation and deep breathing and then hopefully drift into sleep.

Your routine can contain any or all of these, or anything else that you like. The key is that the ritual is relaxing and non-stimulating, and most importantly, consistent. Consistency is that key that will teach your body and mind to start releasing the nighttime chemicals that you need for a restful night's sleep.

Tip #18

Use colors that optimize restfulness

Research has shown that some environments are more conducive to sleep than others. We know that colors can affect our brain and our mood. Avoid bright colors in your room that excite or overstimulate. Stick with soothing colors such as blues (water and sky), neutral colors like ivory or tan, soft calming pastels, or warm natural colors like deep browns and medium greens.

Tip #19

Optimize the temperature

Wear light comfy pj's and avoid heavy quilts that will cause you to be overheated. Research shows that the optimal temperature for sleep is 68 degrees fahrenheit or lower, so preset your thermostat to go to that temperature at night.

Tip #20

Keep it quiet

Make sure your bedroom is completely quiet. If necessary, you can try earplugs, utilize a white noise machine to block out sounds, or use a fan or air purifier to circulate or purify the air while also providing white noise. If you prefer, you can also use a sound machine set to calming noises to help block out sounds while relaxing your body. Popular soothing sounds include the waves, rainfall, or sounds of the forest.

Tip #21

Keep it dark

Keep the lights dim until you are ready to fall asleep and then make the room totally dark to sleep. Make sure curtains block any moonlight or streetlights, and there aren't any glowing lights on electronics visible. If necessary, get blackout curtains and put electronics away in drawers, or use a sleep mask to block out any light.

Tip #22

Utilize scent

Try essential oils that relax. You can use a dispenser, put some on your feet, or drip some on a handkerchief in your pillowcase. You can also put some drops into your bath. Oils that have calming scents include Jasmine, Camomile, Lavender, Sandalwood, and Rose. Experiment to see what works for you.

Tip #23

Try some calming music

There is a reason we play lullabies to babies. Research shows that music decreases cortisol (the stress hormone) and triggers the body to release dopamine (the feel-good hormone). This can boost your mood at bedtime and even help manage pain. Music has been found to decrease the amount of time it takes to fall asleep and improves the quality of the sleep.

Make sure that the music you fall asleep to is slow and relaxing, preferably in the range of 60-80 beats per minute. Check online to find playlists that have been specifically created for helping you fall asleep.

Tip #24

A comfy bed

Make sure that your bed is comfortable, with a mattress and pillow that are supportive. If your mattress is old you might want to consider replacing it. There are also mattress toppers on the market that might make your mattress more comfortable for you. Some people need a firmer mattress and others prefer softer, try some out in the store first to see what works for you. Most stores will allow a period of time when you can use it at home and decide if it works or you need to exchange it. Make sure that you use a supportive pillow that keeps your neck aligned with your spine.

Invest in comfortable bedding that is soft and breathable, and that won't overheat you during the night.

Tip #25

Take a hot bath

A hot bath or even just a warm foot bath before bed has been found to help women fall asleep faster and sleep better (probably men too, but I can't say for sure because only women were used in the study). The water should ideally be 104-109 degrees Fahrenheit, and the bath should take place around 90 minutes before going to sleep. It seems that the hot water actually lowers your body's core temperature , which is a signal to your body that it's time to sleep.

Tip #26

Try this secret drink to make you sleepy

The secret is……. Warm milk and honey! It's the combination of tryptophan and carbohydrates that does it. The tryptophan in the milk induces the body to produce melatonin and the carbs in the honey helps the melatonin deliver to the brain faster. A turkey sandwich will do the same thing (that's why everyone is conked out after Thanksgiving Dinner!) or a banana and milk. But a mug of warm drink is more relaxing and wont force your body to have to work in order to digest.

Tip #27

Try supplemental Melatonin

Our brains naturally produce melatonin when it's dark, which affects our sleep cycle. Taking supplemental melatonin can help you fall asleep naturally without the side effects of a sleep medicine. Keep in mind that although it helps you fall asleep more easily, it's not as effective in helping you stay asleep (which is important to note if your main difficulty is in sleeping through the night ,rather than having difficulty settling down and falling asleep). It's available over the counter but as always ,check with your doctor before starting any new supplements.

Tip # 28

Try an herbal tea

There are a number of herbal teas that have been shown to be effective to improve relaxation and sleep. Chamomile tea is known to have a calming effect on the brain. Valerian tea has been found to make you fall asleep quicker and have a deeper sleep. There are also studies showing Valerian tea helps you sleep for longer, decreases wake ups during the night, and helps with the effects that menopause has on your ability to sleep. There is also a small study showing that if you drink Passionflower tea every night, it improves the quality of sleep. The warmth of a hot tea can alsp help to put you in a more relaxed state.

Tip #29

Try Cognitive Behavioral Therapy

There is a specific type of Cognitive Behavioral Therapy (CBT) that is meant to help with Insomnia, called CBT-i. CBT is usually used for Depression and stress but has been found to be helpful with insomnia by retraining the brain. It has been proven to work in helping people fall asleep faster and have deeper sleep. You can consult a therapist who is trained in CBT, but you can also learn to do it at home.

Tip #30

Check your medicine cabinet

As mentioned earlier, a lot of both prescription medication, over the counter medications, and even natural supplements can have ingre-dients that interfere with sleep.These can include thyroid medicine, beta-blockers, cold medications, some antidepressants, and others. If you think something you are taking is interfering with sleep, talk to your doctor about changing the dosage, time you take it, or alternate formulations of the medication. **Do not just stop taking the medication**

without speaking with your doctor.

Tip #31

Bed only for sleep and sex

Do not eat, study, work, watch TV, talk on the phone, scroll the internet, lie around while awake,or even read in bed. Only use your bed for sleep and sex. If you don't spend your waking time in bed, your brain will make a strong mental connection between being in bed and sleeping. If you spend a lot of awake time in bed it can exacerbate sleep problems. Only get into bed when you are ready to shut the light and go to sleep.

Tip #32

Address any medical issues causing sleep disturbance

If you get muscle cramps, or restless leg syndrome it will wake you up at night and disturb your sleep. There are a number of remedies you can try which people swear are effective, but have not been proven. Speak to your doctor regarding use of these home remedies or the need for possible medication.

If you seem to be sleeping at night but wake up exhausted, or if you snore, you might be experiencing sleep apnea, which are little micro-episodes of stopping breathing when you are sleeping. It is more common in people who are overweight. If you think you are experiencing sleep apnea, speak to your doctor who may order a sleep study and may put you on a nighttime machine called C-PAP, which keeps the airways open and improves breathing during the night. It is an important condition to address because it not only affects your sleep, with all of the ramifications that go with that, but sleep apnea has also been found to be damaging to the heart. Losing weight can often help decrease or fix sleep apnea.

Tip #33

Don't toss and turn

If after 20 minutes you still can't sleep, get out of bed. Staying in bed awake while tossing and turning will just make you anxious and frustrated, and will train your brain to associate being in bed with not sleeping. Instead get out of bed and do something calming like reading, or listening to soft music. Do not use electronics, do not turn on bright lights, do not have a conversation, and do not do anything stimulating, as those things will all make it hard to fall back asleep. As soon as you start feeling a little sleepy, go back to bed.

And for the final tip……

Tip #34

Use the Magic Countdown – 10,3,2,1,0

Here's the daily countdown that is recommended for the best sleep. Try it and see if it helps!

- **Ten** hours before bed: No more caffeine. It takes about 10 hours after you have caffeine for the side effects to go away. This includes soda, coffee, sports drinks, caffeinated teas, chocolate and medications with caffeine.
- **Three** hours before bed: No more food or alcohol. Food will make it hard to fall asleep and alcohol causes waking up in the middle of the night.
- **Two** hours before bed: No more working. It's time to power down and let our body's start transitioning.
- **One** hour before bed: No more electronics. All electronics put out blue light that interferes with melatonin production, which is needed to help regulate the sleep-wake cycle (circadian rhythm).
- **Zero** times you should hit the snooze button in the morning. Break the snooze button habit and get out of bed when the alarm goes off. Pressing snooze repeatedly can have an effect on your ability to fall asleep later that night.

5

Conclusion

So now you have my top 30+ tips to help you fall asleep and have a better quality sleep. I'm hoping that you will utilize them to find that individual magic formula that will give you a good and restful night's sleep on a regular basis.

Good Luck!

I hope this guide was helpful to you. If you like it, I would appreciate it if you could leave a positive review for me on Amazon, Thanks!

Coach Adeena Weiss, PT, MCLC

6

Resources

Suni, E., & Suni, E. (2024, January 10). Healthy sleep habits. Sleep Foundation. https://www.sleepfoundation.org/sleep-habits

The Healthline Editorial Team. (2020, March 29). *Tips to sleep Better.* Healthline. https://www.healthline.com/health/sleep-disorders-prevention#troubleshooting

Count Down–Not Sheep–to a good night's sleep. (2024, February 22).ColumbiaDoctors. https://www.columbiadoctors.org/news/count-down-not-sheep-good-nights-sleep

Nelson, B. (2021, May 25). *Natural sleep remedies that actually work.*The Healthy. https://www.thehealthy.com/sleep/insomnia/insomnia-sleep-remedies/

Mutchler, C. (2024, October 20). *Insomnia facts and statistics: What you need to know.* Verywell Health. https://www.verywellhealth.com/

insomnia-facts-and-statistics-5498718

Adjaye-Gbewonyo, D., Ng, A. E., Black, L. I., U.S. DEPARTMENT OF HEALTH AND HUMAN SERVICES, Centers for Disease Control and Prevention, & National Center for Health Statistics. (2022). Sleep Difficulties in Adults: United States, 2020. In *NCHS Data Brief* (Report No. 436). https://www.cdc.gov/nchs/data/databriefs/db436.pdf

Insomnia - Symptoms and causes. (n.d.). Mayo Clinic. https://www.mayoclinic.org/diseases-conditions/insomnia/symptoms-causes/syc-20355167#:~:text=Insomnia%20may%20be%20the%20main%20problem%20or%20it%20may

Vinall, M. (2021, September 1). *How sleep can affect your hormone levels, plus 12 ways to sleep deep.* Healthline. https://www.healthline.com/health/sleep/how-sleep-can-affect-your-hormone-levels#hormones-and-sleep

Houlton, L. (2024, February 18). *Decluttering a bedroom can improve sleep – experts reveal why.* homesandgardens.com. https://www.homesandgardens.com/solved/decluttering-a-bedroom-can-improve-sleep

Nunez, K. (2024, August 5). *3 Ways to meditate for better sleep.* Healthline. https://www.healthline.com/health/meditation-for-sleep#how-to-meditate

Sleep Foundation. (2023, November 8). *Music and sleep.* https://www.sleepfoundation.org/noise-and-sleep/music#:~:text=Parents%20know%20from%20experience%20that%20%EE%80%80lullabies%EE%80%81

Having trouble sleeping? Try a hot bath before bed. (2019, July 25). *Healthline.* https://www.healthline.com/health-news/having-trouble-sleeping-try-a-hot-bath-before-bed#:~:text=1%20To%20fall%20asleep%20faster%2C%20researchers%20suggest%20taking,to%20the%20body%20that%20it%E2%80%99s%20time%20for%20bed.

Anderson, W. S., MD. (2019). *Dr. A's Habits of Health* (2nd ed.). Habits of Health Press.